alive **Natural Health Guides 8**

William G. Crook MD

Nature's Own
Candida
Cure

Powerful remedies to combat yeast-related health disorders

D0089938

alive **books**

Vancouver
Canada

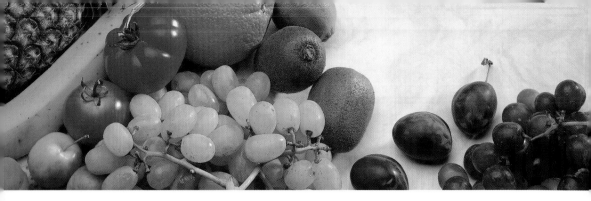

c o n t e n t s

All About Candida

Anti-Candida Recipes

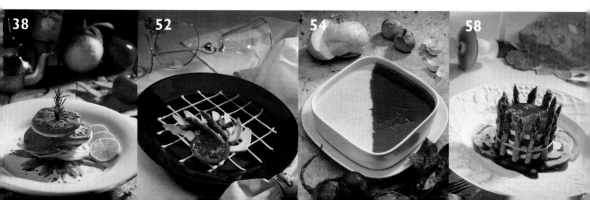

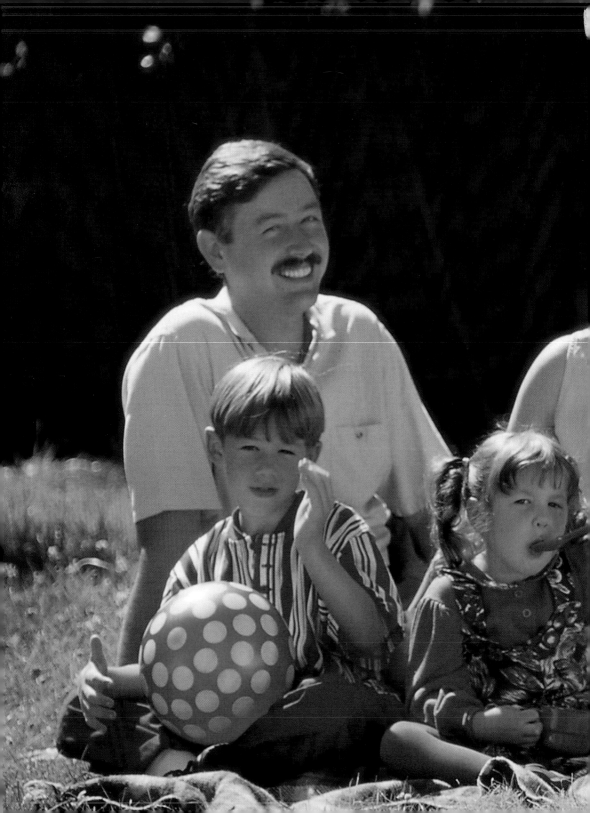

All About Candida

If you feel "sick all over," your health problems may be yeast-connected.

During the past fifteen years I've received thousands of letters and phone calls from people with complaints that focused on a disease or on a particular part of their body. But I've received an even greater number of queries from people who, when asked about their medical history say, "It's hard to know where to begin . . . I feel sick all over."

Three of the most common symptoms in adults with yeast-related health problems are fatigue, headache and depression.

These letters and calls come from men and women of all ages, as well as from parents concerned about their children. These individuals sought help from doctors and specialists, who, in the course of an examination and evaluation, ruled out any number of diseases and disorders. Yet these people still felt sick.

In discussing such situations, Dr. Martin Zwerling and associates have commented:

"Consider the following 'incurable' patient who is being treated by several specialists. Her gynecologist is treating her recurrent vaginitis and irregular menstrual periods while an otolaryngologist is trying to control her external otitis and chronic rhinitis. At the same time, an internist is unsuccessfully attempting to manage symptoms of bloating, indigestion and abdominal pain, and a dermatologist is struggling with bizarre skin rashes, hives and psoriasis.

Lastly, psychiatrists are trying to convince the patient that her nerves are the cause of her extreme irritability, inability to concentrate and depression. We've all been guilty of labeling such patients as 'psychosomatic,' and since there is 'nothing physically wrong,' conclude that we cannot cure them. Incurable? Not if you think yeast. This patient and thousands like her are suffering from chronic candidiasis."

The Yeast Connection . . . .

The relationship of yeast infections to chronic illness was first described by Orian C. Truss MD, more than twenty years ago. However, because he published his observations in a non-peer reviewed journal, most physicians were unaware of them. Truss's observations spread to the public through magazine articles and television programs, including Cable News Network (CNN) and

The Phil Donahue Show. As a result, the public learned about yeast-related health problems before scientific studies were published in major medical journals.

Three of the most common symptoms in adults with yeast-related health problems are fatigue, headache and depression. However, symptoms of systemic candidiasis are varied and diverse, and typically manifest themselves in five areas of the body:

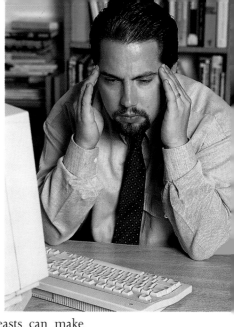

Since the first edition of my book, *The Yeast Connection Handbook*, was published in 1984, critics have been asking for "scientific" proof. They want to see double-blind studies; they want to be able to quantify my claim that yeasts can make people sick. In response to these challenges I began knocking on

Common Candida Symptoms	
Digestive System	Symptoms include bloating, gas, cramps, and diarrhea alternating with constipation.
Nervous System	Symptoms include abnormal fatigue, anxiety, mood swings, memory loss, depression, insomnia and mental fogginess. In children, autism, hyperactivity and learning disabilities may be indications of candidiasis.
Skin	Symptoms include hives, psoriasis, eczema, excessive sweating, acne and nail infections.
Genito-urinary Tract	In women, common symptoms include PMS (depression, mood swings fluid retention, cramps) recurrent bladder or vaginal infections and a loss of interest in sex. In males, common problems include chronic rectal or anal itching, recurrent prostatitis, impotence, and genital rashes.
Endocrine System	The thyroid, adrenal glands and the pancreas may be affected by candida. Symptoms include fatigue, weakness, low body temperature, constipation and sugar craving.

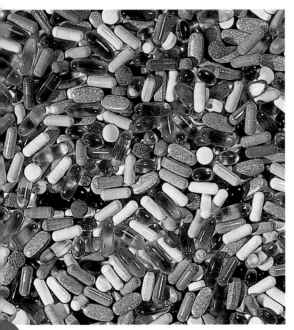

Many of those being treated by several specialists, and taking a number of prescriptions as a result, may have to start thinking "yeast."

doors, urging medical institutions such as the National Institute of Health to look into the relationship between yeast infections and chronic illnesses. My pleas fell on deaf ears.

Times have changed, and an increasing number of traditional physicians have made observations that support the connection between candidiasis and chronic illness. Still, the battle is fought at the frontlines—in the doctor's office—where patients look for relief from yeast-related illnesses. And candidiasis is not an easy call.

Current laboratory tests do not enable a physician to make a diagnosis of a yeast-related illness. Instead, the diagnosis must be based on clinical observations, which requires diligence and commitment on the part of the physician.

According to an editorial by John Bennett MD, in the *New England Journal of Medicine*, few illnesses have sparked as much hostility between the medical community and the lay public as the chronic candidiasis syndrome: "Those who argue for the existence of this complex of symptoms...have leveled a serious charge against the medical community, claiming it is not filling one of its most important obligations to its patients. The charge is simply put: You physicians are not listening to your patients."

Are Your Health Problems Yeast Connected? . . . .

The common yeast *Candida albicans* has been linked to conditions such as eczema, psoriasis, acne and sinusitis, as well as to lupus, rheumatoid arthritis and multiple sclerosis.

I'm not saying that *Candida albicans* is the cause of all these problems. But candida may be one of the causes—even a major cause—of these and other health problems.

The Candida Quiz

To help you determine if your health problems are connected to yeast, answer the following questions. If you answer "yes" to any question, circle the number in the right-hand column. When you've completed the questionnaire, add up the numbers you've circled.

	Yes	No	Score
1. Have you taken repeated or prolonged courses of anti-bacterial drugs?	☐	☐	**4**
2. Have you been bothered by recurrent vaginal, prostate or urinary infections?	☐	☐	**3**
3. Do you feel "sick all over," yet the cause has not been found?	☐	☐	**2**
4. Are you bothered by hormone disturbances, including PMS, menstrual irregularities, sexual dysfunction, sugar craving, low body temperature or fatigue?	☐	☐	**2**
5. Are you unusually sensitive to tobacco smoke, perfumes, colognes and other chemical odors?	☐	☐	**2**
6. Are you bothered by memory or concentration problems? Do you sometimes feel "spaced out?"	☐	☐	**2**
7. Have you taken prolonged courses of prednisone or other steroids; or have you taken birth control pills for more than three years?	☐	☐	**2**
8. Do some foods disagree with you or trigger your symptoms?	☐	☐	**1**
9. Do you suffer with constipation, diarrhea, bloating and abdominal pain?	☐	☐	**1**
10. Does your skin itch, tingle or burn; or is it unusually dry; or are you bothered by rashes?	☐	☐	**1**

Scoring for women: If your score is 9 or more, your health problems are probably yeast-connected. If your score is 12 or more, your health problems are almost certainly yeast-connected.
Scoring for men: If your score is 7 or more, your health problems are probably yeast-connected. If your score is 10 or more, your health problems are almost certainly yeast-connected.

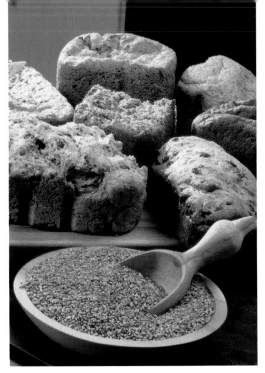

Not all yeasts are bad. The yeast used to leaven bread, for example, is harmless.

What are Yeasts? . . .

Yeasts are single-cell organisms that live on the surfaces of all living things, including fruits, vegetables, grains and your skin. Yeast is a kind of fungus. Mildew, mold, monilia and candida are all names that are used to describe different types of yeast. One particular type of yeast, *Candida albicans*, normally lives on the inner warm creases and crevices of your digestive tract and vagina.

Candida growth is kept in balance by so-called "good bacteria" including Lactobacillus acidophilus and Bifidobacterium bifidum, and by your immune system. However, candida is an opportunistic organism, and if the immune system is compromised the tenuous balance is upset and the good bacteria are destroyed. Candida then multiplies, and the resulting overgrowth can lead to health problems, which affect many parts of your body.

Not all yeasts are bad. In fact, of the thousands of existing species of yeast, only a small percentage can survive in the human body, and of these, only a few can induce disease.

Most yeasts, such as those used to leaven bread and brew beer, are harmless. Moreover, there are numerous yeast-based supplements, such as nutritional yeast and Floradix Iron Yeast Extract, that promote good health. *Candida albicans*, however, has a Dr. Jeckyl and Mr. Hyde type of personality: it has the ability to change from a single-cell yeast into a branching fungal form, able to burrow beneath the surfaces of the mucous membranes. Thus, if not kept in check by a healthy diet and a well-functioning immune system, candida can become a threat to your health.

Good vs. Bad Yeast

Not all yeasts are bad. Of the thousands of existing species of yeast, only a small percentage can induce disease.

Factors that Promote Yeast Overgrowth . . .

Like all fungi, *Candida albicans* thrives in warm, moist areas. Under normal conditions, candida exists within us in a healthy balance, and the body's immune system keeps it from spreading. When your immune system is strong, candida yeasts present no problem. But, if you take broad-spectrum antibiotics or other medications (the birth control pill or cortisone, for example) the good bacteria that prevent fungal infections from developing are knocked out. The candida yeasts are not affected, so they multiply and put out toxins that further weaken the immune system. Consequently, you may experience repeated infections, and these infections may be treated with another round of antibiotics, encouraging further growth of candida...and so a vicious cycle develops. While there may be many factors that contribute to feeling "sick all over," I am convinced that it is repeated courses of broad-spectrum antibiotics that are the main "villain."

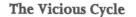

The Vicious Cycle

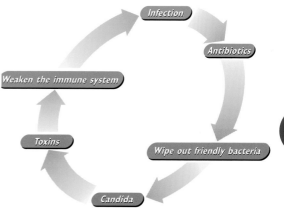

A yeast infection in one part of your body can cause symptoms elsewhere in several different ways. Candida overgrowth in your intestine may create what is called a "leaky gut," an inflammation of the intestinal wall that results in substances permeating the protective lining of the gut. Consequently, toxins and food allergens can pass easily through this membrane and travel to other parts of your body.

Yeast and the Immune System . . . . . .

Your immune system is composed of many different defenders, including white blood cells, antibodies and immunoglobulins. Some "sit" just under the surface of your mucous membranes–ready to pounce on invaders. Others circulate and patrol the deeper tissues and organs of the body, attacking and wiping out enemies that may have sneaked in.

When your immune system is weak you are apt to develop yeast and/or fungus infections of the skin, nails or vagina. You may also become more susceptible to viral, bacterial and other infections, and develop mold, chemical, food and other allergies, intolerances and sensitivities.

Nutritional deficiencies caused by inadequate intake and/or poor absorption of essential nutrients also weaken the immune system. So does living or working in an environment loaded with pollutants. A heavy load of environmental molds also adversely affects your immune system. So does emotional stress.

Yeast toxins affect the immune system, the nervous system and the endocrine system. Moreover, these systems are all connected. So, yeast toxins play a role in causing allergies, vaginal, bladder, prostate and other infections, as well as headaches, fatigue, depression and other nervous symptoms. They also play an important role in causing disturbances of hormone function, including loss of sexual interest, impotence, premenstrual tension, menstrual irregularities, infertility and pelvic pain.

Health Problems in Women . . . .

Of those individuals who develop yeast-related health problems, approximately 85 percent will be women.

Women develop yeast-related problems more often than men, and pre-menopausal women appear to be especially susceptible. There appear to be several reasons for this:
• Hormonal changes associated with the menstrual cycle promote yeast growth, as do birth control pills and pregnancy.
• The anatomical characteristics of women make them more susceptible to vaginitis and urinary tract infections.
• Women visit physicians more often then men. Accordingly, they are more apt to receive antibiotics for health complaints.

Health Problems in Men . . . .

Men also suffer from yeast-related health disorders. The following list of symptoms may indicate a problem with yeast.
• Crave and consume lots of sweets, bread and alcohol.

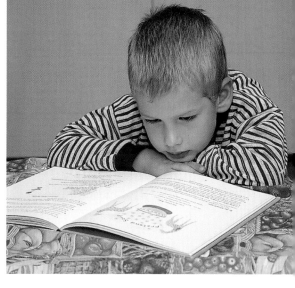

- Bothered by persistent jock itch, athlete's foot or fungus infection of the nails.
- Troubled by food and inhalant allergies.
- Complain of fatigue, depression and nervousness.
- Recurrent digestive problems.
- Bothered by dampness, chemicals or tobacco.
- Impaired sex drive.
- Partner has a yeast problem.

Health Problems in Children . . . .

As a pediatrician I'm interested in the problems that affect millions of infants, young children and teenagers. I'm especially concerned about recurrent ear disorders, behavioral and learning problems, and juvenile delinquency.

These problems are increasing in frequency and current methods of management appear to be ineffective. These problems are often yeast-related.

Repeated courses of antibiotics given for childhood ear infections set up a vicious cycle of recurrent infections.

13

Breaking the Cycle . . . .

In my opinion, repeated antibiotics given for ear infections set up a vicious cycle, which includes recurrent infections and nervous symptoms of various types. Here are my recommendations for breaking the vicious cycle of ear infections and preventing the development of hyperactivity, attention deficits and autism:

1. Don't rush to your physician and ask for an antibiotic when your infant or young child complains of mild ear pain. Instead, use simple herbal remedies to relieve discomfort, such as a warm chamomile infusion to wash the ears. There are also several homeopathic remedies that may be effective, including *Belladona*, *Ferrum phosphoricum*, *Chamomilla* and *Pulsatilla*. The choice of a remedy will depend on the

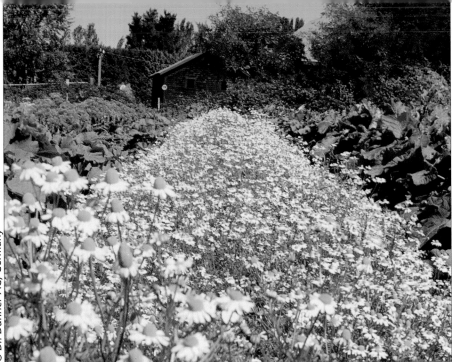

Many homeopathic remedies, including Chamomilla, may be helpful in treating ear infections in children, therefore eliminating the need for an antibiotic.

symptoms your child exhibits. Consult a homeopath or your health care practioner. There are also several excellent books on the subject.

2. Change your child's diet. Eliminate all sugar-containing foods and beverages, as well as milk and dairy products. In their place, offer whole foods, bottled or filtered water and fresh squeezed orange juice.

3. When your child develops a respiratory infection, give extra vitamin C. You can purchase vitamin C crystals or powder from a health food store. Add one teaspoon to six ounces of water. Offer one-half to one ounce of this mixture every one to three hours, unless it causes a stomach ache or loose stools.

4. Purchase liquid zinc sulfate from your health food store or pharmacy. When taken along with vitamin C it strengthens the immune system. Give your child one to two milligrams four times a day.

5. If your physician examines your child and suggests an antibiotic for an ear or other infections, ask him/her if your child can get along without the antibiotic.

6. If your child is given an antibiotic, ask your physician to prescribe oral nystatin powder. Give your child 250,000 units

(approximately 1/16 teaspoon) by mouth with each dose of an antibiotic. I do not recommend Mycostatin or Nilstat suspension as they are sweetened with sugar.

7. Go to your health food store or pharmacy and ask for a probiotic powder or capsule. These products contain *Lactobacillus acidophilus* and other helpful bacteria. Give your child one capsule or one-quarter teaspoon of the powder with each dose of the antibiotic.

8. After the course of antibiotics has been completed, I recommend continuing the nystatin and probiotic in the same amounts, two or three times daily for one or more weeks. Nystatin discourages the growth of yeast in the intestinal tract and the probiotics replace the important friendly bacteria. These products help heal the "leaky gut," lessen the absorption of milk, wheat and other allergens, and decrease the chance of your child developing repeated ear problems.

Most people with yeast-related health problems resemble the proverbial overburdened camel.

Regaining your Health . . . .

The Road to Recovery

Candida isn't like a dragon that you can slay with a single thrust of a sword or kill with a magic bullet. Most people with yeast-related health problems resemble the proverbial overburdened camel. To regain your health you will need to unload many bundles of straw. This may take months–even a year or more. But then your camel can get on her feet and start walking–then running. You can overcome your health problems and get your life back on track!

Believe in Yourself

Believing that you have some control over your condition is an essential first step. You do not need to feel victimized by candida; you can make the changes necessary for better health.

Take Charge

The second step is taking charge. Read, study and learn. Be responsible. Although you will need help from kind and caring health professionals, you must make the major decisions.

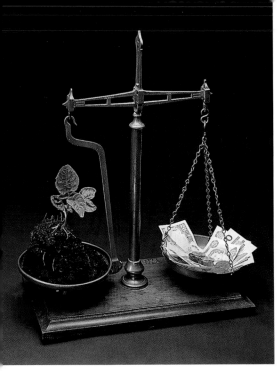

A clean environment is not only essential for health, it's priceless.

Control Exposure to Chemicals

Almost without exception, every person with a yeast-related disorder is made worse by exposure to chemicals. According to an article published in the *Journal of the American Medical Association* (*JAMA*), the risks from industrial pollutants dumped or leaked into the environment are "less than the risk from exposures in the home, such as smoking, showering, using room deodorizers and storing and wearing dry-cleaned clothes." So, begin at once to get rid of the chemical pollutants in your home.

Numerous studies have shown that chemical exposure adversely affects the immune system. The more chemicals you're exposed to, the greater your chances of developing health problems. Here are some things you can do to lessen the chances that chemicals may be contributing to your health problems.

Don't smoke or let other people smoke in your home. People in homes where others are smoking experience twice as many respiratory infections and other health problems as individuals in smoke-free homes. Moreover, such infections set up a vicious cycle of other health problems.

Don't spray insecticides in your home. You should also store insecticides, paint thinners and other toxic chemicals in an outside shed or garage. Don't keep them under the kitchen sink or in the basement where fumes can leak into the house.

Buy all natural fibers. If you buy permanent press clothing or sheets, wash them before using.

Air dry-cleaned items. Remove dry-cleaned items from their plastic wraps and thoroughly air them outside before bringing them into your house.

Avoid odorous and potentially toxic substances in your home. These include paints, formaldehyde, gas stoves and many perfumes and colognes.

Get an air purifier to remove dust, molds and some chemicals.

Have your home tested for the presence of toxic substances. If you suspect that your home is contaminated from pesticides and/or other chemicals have a professional test for dangerous levels of toxins.

Nutritional Supplements

Many health professionals with impeccable scientific credentials have noted the importance of nutritional supplements. But supplements are not nutrient substitutes; it is essential that you eat a healthy, balanced diet. However, getting optimal amounts of vitamins and minerals usually requires supplementing the diet. For my adult patients with yeast-related health problems, I prescribe the following supplements to be taken daily: (Note: These suggested amounts may vary considerably from those prescribed by your health care practitioner, who will take into account your specific medical profile.)

> **Supplements are not nutrients; it is essential that you eat a healthy, balanced diet.**

Daily Supplements for Adults with Yeast-Related Health Problems

Vitamin A	5,000-10,000 IU	Vitamin E	400-600 IU
Beta-carotene	15,000 IU	Calcium	500 mgs
Vitamin B1	25-100 mgs	Magnesium	500 mgs
Vitamin B2	50 mgs	Inositol	100 mgs
Niacin	50 mgs	Citrus bioflavonoids	100 mgs
Niacinamide	100-150 mgs	PABA	50 mgs
Pantothenic acid	100-500 mgs	Zinc	15-30 mgs
Vitamin B6	25-100 mgs	Copper	1-2 mgs
Folic acid	200-800 mcgs	Manganese	20 mgs
Vitamin B12	100-2,000 mcgs	Selenium	100-200 mcgs
Biotin	300 mcgs	Chromium	200 mcgs
Choline (Bitartrate)	100 mgs	Molybdenum	100 mcgs
Vitamin C	1,000-10,000 mgs	Vanadium	25 mcgs
Vitamin D	400-800 IU	Boron	1 mg

Essential Fatty Acids (EFAs)

Our bodies are composed of billions of cells of various sizes, shapes and functions. A membrane composed of special types of fats called essential fatty acids, or EFAs, surrounds each cell. These "good" fats come directly and only from food and they have many diverse functions.

During the past decade, almost without exception, physicians treating patients with yeast-related health problems

Physicians routinely use essential fatty acid supplements as part of a candida treatment program. have used EFA supplements as a part of their treatment program.

There are two general classes of EFAs: the omega-3 fatty acids and the omega-6 fatty acids. Omega 6 essential fatty acids are found in primrose, safflower and sunflower oils; omega-3 is abundant only in flax seed and some fish oils. We have doubled our intake of omega-6 but decreased omega-3 intake to one-sixth of what we used to get in traditional diets. In order to rectify this imbalance, I recommend taking flax oil: The usual dose is one to two tablespoons a day. You can mix it with lemon juice and use it as a salad dressing, or you can take it straight. Because flax oil can become rancid, it should be dispensed in dark glass bottles and kept refrigerated. The bottles should also be dated, as it has a short shelf life, three to four months at most. You will find flax oil in health food stores. For a more detailed look at flax and essential fatty acids see *Fantastic Flax* and *Good Fats and Oils*, both are titles in the *alive* Natural Health Guides series.

The Candida Diet . . . .

This is the most involved step in your road to recovery, and it will probably require a major shift in your shopping and eating habits. In this section, I have outlined what foods to avoid and what you should replace them with, as well as steps to take to implement dietary changes. (Note: You will find a more complete listing of food items at the back of this book.)

Purge the Pantry
Go to your kitchen, pantry and refrigerator and *get rid of sugar,* corn syrup, white bread and other white-flour products, soda pop, most ready-to-eat cereals, and all sugar- and fat-laden snack foods. Foods and beverages containing these nutritionally deficient simple carbohydrates encourage yeast overgrowth and promote poor health. To overcome your candida-related health

problems you'll need to avoid them. Get rid of processed and prepared junk foods, which have hydrogenated or partially hydrogenated fats, food coloring and additives.

Shop mainly around the outer edges of your supermarket. Look for fresh and frozen vegetables; fresh meat, poultry, fish, seafood and eggs; olive oil and pure butter. I especially recommend organically grown foods, as they haven't been chemically contaminated. You'll find these foods in many health food stores and in some supermarkets.

Eat Freely
Eggs and fish.
Low carbohydrate vegetables: Cruciferous vegetables (e.g., broccoli, cauliflower, cabbage) carrots, lettuce, onion, peppers.

Eat Sparingly
High carbohydrate vegetables: Potatoes, squash, beets, avocado, beans, peas and other legumes.
Whole grains (non-enriched): Wheat, brown rice, corn, oats, barley.
Grain alternatives: Buckwheat, quinoa, amaranth.

Avoid
Sugar and foods containing sugar.
Packaged foods.
Processed and smoked meats.
Mushrooms and truffles.
Most condiments and sauces.
Fruit (during the first three weeks).
Leftovers (Leftovers should be frozen immediately, as molds are quick to grow in them).

Drink Freely
Water: Drink eight glasses of water a day. Ordinary tap water, however, may be contaminated with lead, bacteria or parasites. I recommend bottled spring water or distilled water. Green tea provides many health benefits.

Drink Sparingly
Coffee: If you can't get along without your coffee, limit your intake to one to two cups a day. Drink it plain.

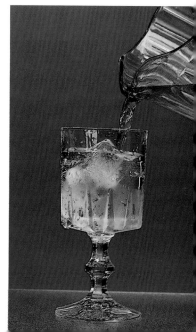

Avoid

Fruit juices: Fruit juices are high in fructose, a type of sugar.

Alcoholic beverages: Wines, beers and other alcoholic beverages contain large amounts of quick-acting carbohydrates.

Diet drinks: These beverages possess no nutritional value, and contain ingredients that may disagree with sensitive individuals.

Implementing the diet

To begin the candida diet, avoid sugar (in all its forms) and other quick-acting carbohydrates. Canned, bottled, boxed and other packaged and processed foods usually contain refined sugar products and other hidden ingredients. You'll not only need to avoid these sugar-containing foods during the early weeks of your diet, you'll need to avoid them indefinitely.

Most people with candida-related illnesses can, as they improve, follow a less rigid diet.

For the first ten days of your diet, avoid foods containing yeast. The following is a list of foods that contain yeasts or molds.

- Breads, pastries and other raised bakery goods.
- All cheeses (especially moldy cheeses, such as Roquefort).
- Condiments, sauces and foods containing vinegar.
- Malt products (malted milk drinks, cereals and candy).
- Processed and smoked meats.
- Edible fungi (all types of mushrooms, morels and truffles).
- Melons (watermelon, honeydew melon and, especially, cantaloupe).
- Dried and candied fruits (raisins, apricots, dates, prunes, figs, pineapple).
- Leftovers (molds grows quickly in leftover food).

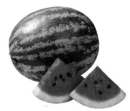

Test Your Yeast Tolerance

After you've avoided yeast-containing foods for ten days, you can find out if you're sensitive to yeast by eating a tablet of brewer's yeast, which you can get at a health food store. If it doesn't bother you, eat some moldy cheese. If consuming these yeasty foods triggers symptoms, stay away from them for several weeks, and then experiment further.

Truly yeast-free diets are impossible to come by because you'll find yeast and molds on the surfaces of all fruits, vegetables and grains. Once you've found out that you're sensitive to yeast, you'll need to be your own judge as to how well you tolerate food that may contain yeasts or molds.

The Fruit Challenge

Avoid fruit during the first three weeks of your diet. The sugars in fruits, although combined with fiber, are more quickly released and may trigger yeast overgrowth. But, to see if they bother you, you can do the fruit challenge. Here's how:

Take a small bite of banana. Ten minutes later, eat a second bite. If no reaction occurs in the next hour, eat the whole banana. If you tolerate the banana without developing symptoms try strawberries, pineapple or apple the next day. If you show no symptoms after these fruit challenges, chances are you can eat fruit in moderation. But feel your way along; don't overdo it.

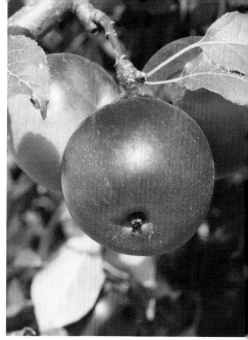

Take the time to figure out what, if any, fruit triggers symptoms related to yeast overgrowth.

21

If your health problems are yeast-connected, you may improve—often dramatically—when you stop eating foods containing significant amounts of cane sugar, beet sugar, corn syrup, fructose, dextrose or honey. Then if you follow other parts of the candida-control program you may find that after two or three months you can consume foods that contain small amounts of sugar.

However, if you are allergic to yeasts and molds, you may pay for any dietary infraction. And you may not achieve maximum improvement until you avoid all foods that contain yeasts and molds. If you are still experiencing problems, you'll need to carry out food allergy detective work. In so doing, you identify and avoid all foods that cause adverse or allergic reactions. Common offenders include milk, egg, wheat, corn and soy, although any food can be a troublemaker.

Each person differs. You are unique. In following the candida diet, use a trial and error approach. Most of my patients with candida-related illnesses can, as they improve, follow a less rigid diet—especially if they are taking other steps to regain their health.

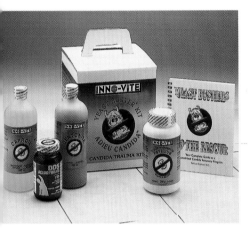

Antiyeast Medications

If your health problems are yeast-related, changing your diet is an important step toward good health. Prescription antifungal medications are an equally important step. Such medications are effective in "knocking out" or limiting the growth of yeast organisms, including *Candida albicans*. As is the case with other prescription drugs, they may, in rare cases, cause significant adverse reactions. However, based on the observations of physicians who have used them in treating thousands of patients, they are remarkably safe and highly effective.

Health stores offer a Yeast Buster Kit, which includes four effective products: Psyllium, caproil, bentonite and DDS acidophilus powder.

My long-time favorite prescription treatment is nystatin. One of its outstanding features is its safety. Although it knocks out yeast on contact, it works only in the intestine and very little is absorbed into the bloodstream.

Which medication (or medications) should you take? How long should you take it? These decisions will, of course, be made by your own physician, and will be based on the duration of your health problems and his/her experiences and preferences.

Die-Off Reactions

A word about "die-off" reactions: Many people who take nystatin or other prescription or nonprescription anti-yeast medications feel worse before feeling better. This is a result of "die-off" reactions. As the candida organisms are killed off, the body is flooded with toxins from the ruptured yeast cells. The body immediately reacts with an inflammatory immune response that can cause fatigue, depression, irritability, aches and

---

Natural Yeast Fighters

There are a number of foods that have antifungal properties. Among the most potent are garlic, onion, green onion, radish, black radish and horseradish. Garlic and onion are particularly beneficial, especially if eaten raw. And radish, horseradish and watercress contain oils that suppress the growth of the candida yeast. Add fresh watercress to your salad; not only does it taste delicious but it aids in the fight against *Candida albicans*.

abdominal pain. It may take a few days (or longer) for your body to get rid of the dead yeast products, but you will begin to feel better.

Nonprescription Anti-Yeast Medications

There are also nonprescription substances and products that help limit or retard the growth of candida in the digestive tract. Among my favorite remedies are probiotics, caprylic acid and citrus seed extracts.

Probiotics

Probiotics are a group of friendly bacteria–including *Lactobacillus acidophilus* and *Bifidum bacterium*–that contribute to our health. Although they are not potent agents for "knocking out" yeasts, recent reports indicate that they do help. I recommend probiotics as a nutritional supplement for all my patients.

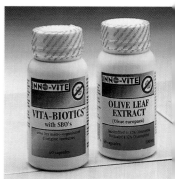

Ask your natural health care practitioner about products to help control candida.

Caprylic acid

Caprylic acid, a naturally occurring fatty acid, has been found to have antifungal properties and to be effective in controlling candida in the intestinal tract. Some health care professionals feel that it is just as effective as nystatin. Although caprylic acid products discourage the growth of *Candida albicans* in the intestinal tract, they are no "cure-all." Their use should be supervised by a health professional.

Citrus Seed Extract

Like nystatin and caprylic acid, this antifungal agent discourages the growth of *Candida albicans* in the intestinal tract and is thought to be highly effective. Particularly recommended is Tricyclene, a product that combines grapefruit seed extract and the herbs artemesia and berberine.

Other products used to control candida include garlic, olive leaf extract, goldenseal, aloe vera and Kolorex, a New Zealand herbal product. Research these and other products and discuss their usage with your health care practitioner.

Exercise

Whether or not your health problems are related to yeast, you will need to exercise if you want to enjoy good health. Exercise will increase your energy level, mental alertness and feeling of

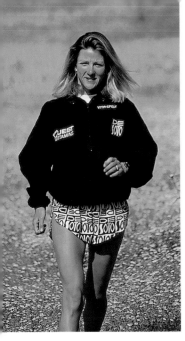

well-being. Furthermore, studies have shown that people who exercise develop fewer illnesses and are less apt to have accidents.

Aerobic exercises, which require the use of oxygen to produce energy, are especially effective. Recommended aerobic exercises include walking, running, aerobic dance, swimming, cross-country skiing, bicycling and rowing. If you want to look good, feel good and overcome health problems of any sort, you'll need to exercise regularly.

Lifestyle Changes

If your health problems are yeast-related, it will help to change your diet, get rid of chemical pollutants in your home and take antiyeast medications and nutritional supplements. But there are other things that you can do, too. In his comprehensive book *Staying Healthy with Nutrition*, Elson M. Haas, MD, lists eighty-eight survival suggestions, including these lifestyle changes:

- Avoid excessive sun exposure. With the depletion of the ozone layer and the effect of ultraviolet light, the risks outweigh the benefits.
- Practice some sort of stress reduction daily. Meditate, or breathe deeply and relax for at least fifteen to twenty minutes.
- Reduce or avoid alcohol use. Alcohol depresses the senses and reduces immune resistance.
- Avoid habitual drug use, such as consumption of caffeine in coffee, tea or colas.
- Drink more clean water. Drink less soda, coffee and juice.
- Wear more natural-fiber clothes (cotton, rayon and silk), especially if you are sensitive to synthetic materials.
- Buy and use organic foods, those grown without chemicals, fertilizers and pesticides.
- Take antioxidant nutrients.
- Eat more cruciferous vegetables and rotate foods to avoid allergic/sensitivity reactions.
- If possible, use natural or full spectrum lights at work.
- Take regular breaks from a computer—walk and stretch, drink some water and get fresh air.

The Mind/Body Connection

Although I was aware that psychological factors could contribute to health, I didn't really pay much attention to them until recently. At a meeting of the American Holistic Medical Association, I heard many fascinating discussions on the mind/body connection, including presentations from Drs. Larry Dossey, Deepak Chopra and James Gordon. On returning home, I began to read books that dealt with the relationship of psychological stimuli to physical symptoms. The authors invariably attested to the value of meditation, visualization, hypnosis, biofeedback and relaxation techniques in the prevention and treatment of a variety of illnesses.

Food Allergies and Sensitivities

Unusual reactions to substances in a person's diet or environment have been recognized for thousands of years. But it wasn't until 1906 that the word "allergy" was coined by the Austrian pediatrician Clemens von Pirquet. He put together two Greek words–*allos*, meaning "other" and *ergon*, meaning "action." To von Pirquet allergy meant altered reactivity.

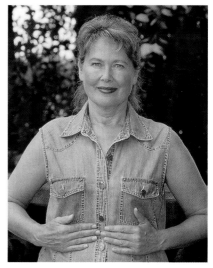

Some doctors feel that the term allergy should be limited to those conditions for which an immunological response can be demonstrated using allergy skin tests or more sophisticated laboratory tests. But other conscientious physicians feel that the allergic and hypersensitivity diseases are much broader in scope, and note the unreliability of food skin tests and the value of trial elimination diets.

Tracking Down Your Hidden Food Sensitivities

Almost without exception, every person with a yeast-related problem is bothered by food sensitivities. To identify the foods that may be contributing to your symptoms, you must carefully plan and properly execute an elimination/challenge diet.

The diet is divided into two parts: First, you'll need to eliminate a number of your usual foods to see if your symptoms

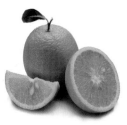

improve or disappear. Then, in five to ten days, when your symptoms show marked improvement, eat the eliminated foods again—introducing one food per day—and see which ones cause symptoms. Keep a record of your symptoms in a notebook:

a) For three days (or more) before beginning the diet.

b) While following the elimination part of the diet (five to ten days).

c) While reintroducing the eliminated foods (one food per day).

During the first two to four days of the diet you're apt to feel irritable, hungry and tired. You may develop a headache or leg cramps. If the foods you have eliminated are causing your symptoms, you'll usually feel better by the fourth, fifth or sixth day of the diet. Almost always, improvement is felt by the tenth day.

After you're certain that you feel better, and your improvement has lasted for at least two days, begin adding foods back to your diet—one per day. If you are allergic to one or more of the eliminated foods, you will most likely develop headache, fatigue or other symptoms when you introduce the foods again. These symptoms will usually appear within a few minutes to a few hours. However, sometimes you may not notice the symptoms until the next day.

After you have completed the elimination part of your diet, add the following foods to your diet, one food per day, and make note of any reactions. Make sure you have the foods in their pure form. Following are suggestions:

> Egg: Soft-boiled, or scrambled in pure butter or coconut butter.
>
> Citrus: Peel an orange and eat it.
>
> Milk: Use whole milk.
>
> Wheat: Cream of wheat cereal or Shredded Wheat.
>
> Food coloring: Buy a set of food dyes. Mix several colors in a glass; add a teaspoon of that mixture to a glass of water and sip on it.
>
> Chocolate: Use Baker's cooking chocolate or a pure cocoa powder. You can sweeten it with maple syrup.
>
> Corn: Use fresh corn on the cob or pure corn syrup.
>
> Sugar: Use natural cane sugar (Sucanat® or Rapadura™).

Most people with yeast-related health problems also have food sensitivities.

Other Suggestions

- Plan ahead. Don't start your diet the week before Christmas or on some other holiday.
- Don't start the diet when you're traveling or visiting friends or relatives.
- Reintroduce the foods you least suspect first.
- Save the foods you suspect are troublemakers until last.
- Eat a small portion of the eliminated food for breakfast. If you show no reaction, eat more of the food in two hours and again in four hours. In six hours, eat a lot of it. If you show no reaction, that food isn't causing problems.
- Keep the rest of your diet the same while carrying out the challenges.
- If you think you develop symptoms when you add a food, don't eat more of that food. Wait until the reaction subsides (usually 24 to 48 hours) before you add another food.
- If you find that a food causes your symptoms, keep it out of your diet for three to four weeks, then try it again. Many food-sensitive people find that they can eat a small amount of the food every four to seven days.

By eliminating the foods that you suspect to be troublesome, and then closely monitoring your reaction to them upon reintroduction, you will discover what foods you should avoid. And this, combined with the other steps outlined in this book, should put you on the road to recovery from your yeast-connected health problems.

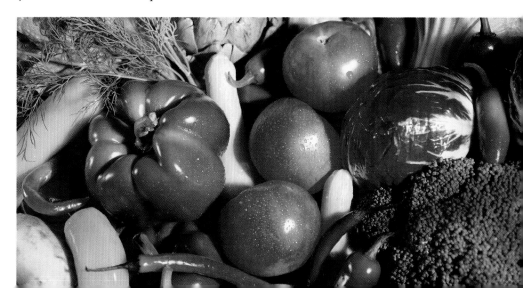

Candida Questionnaire

If you would like to know if your health problems are yeast-related take this comprehensive test. Questions in Section A focus on your medical history—factors that promote the growth of *Candida albicans* and that are frequently found in people with yeast-related health problems. In Section B you'll find a list of 23 symptoms that are often present in patients with yeast-related health problems. Section C consists of 33 other symptoms that are sometimes seen in people with yeast-related problems—yet they may also be found in people with other disorders.

Filling out and scoring the questionnaire should help you and your physician evaluate the possible role that *Candida albicans* play in your health problems. It will not, however, give a definitive yes or no answer.

Section A: History

1. Have you ever taken tetracycline, or other antibiotics, for acne for one month or longer? 35
2. Have you, at any time in your life, taken broad-spectrum antibiotics or other antibacterial medication for respiratory, urinary or other infections for two months or longer, or in shorter courses four or more times in a one-year period? 35
3. Have you taken a broad-spectrum antibiotic drug—even in a single dose? 6
4. Have you at any time in your life been bothered by persistent prostatitis, vaginitis or other problems affecting your reproductive organs? 25
5. Are you bothered by memory or concentration problems—do you sometimes feel spaced out? 20
6. Do you feel "sick all over," yet despite visits to many different physicians the cause has not been found? 20
7. Have you been pregnant?
    Two or more times? 5
    One time? 3
8. Have you taken birth control pills?
    For more than two years 15
    For six months to two years 8
9. Have you taken steroids orally, by injection or inhalation?
    For more than two weeks 15
    For two weeks or less 6
10. Does exposure to perfume, insecticides, fabric shop odors and other chemicals provoke symptoms?
    Moderate to severe 20
    Mild 5
11. Does tobacco smoke really bother you? 10

12. Are your symptoms worse on damp, muggy days or in moldy places? .. 20
13. Have you had athlete's foot, ring worm, jock itch or other chronic fungal infections of the skin or nails?
    Severe or persistent 20
    Mild to moderate 10
14. Do you crave sugar? 10

Total Score, Section A _____

Section B: Major Symptoms

For each of your symptoms, enter the appropriate figure in the point score column.

If a symptom is occasional or mild	3 points
If a symptom is frequent and/or moderately severe	6 points
If a symptom is severe and/or disabling	9 points

Add total score and record it at the end of this section.

- Fatigue or lethargy _____
- Feeling of being "drained" _____
- Depression or manic depression _____
- Numbness, burning or tingling _____
- Headache _____
- Muscle aches _____
- Muscle weakness or paralysis _____
- Pain and/or swelling in joints _____
- Abdominal pain _____
- Constipation and/or diarrhea _____
- Bloating, belching or intestinal gas _____
- Troublesome vaginal burning, itching or discharge _____
- Prostatitis _____
- Impotence _____
- Loss of sexual desire or feeling _____
- Endometriosis or infertility _____
- Cramps and/or other menstrual irregularities _____
- Premenstrual tension _____
- Attacks of anxiety or crying _____
- Cold hands or feet, low body temperature _____
- Hypothyroidism _____
- Shaking or irritable when hungry _____
- Cystitis or interstitial cystitis _____

Total Score, Section B _____

Section C: Other Symptoms

For each of your symptoms, enter the appropriate figure in the point score column.

If a symptom is occasional or mild	1 point
If a symptom is frequent and/or moderately severe	2 points
If a symptom is severe and/or disabling	3 points

Add total score and record it at the end of this section.

- Drowsiness, including inappropriate drowsiness _____
- Irritability _____
- Incoordination _____
- Frequent mood swings _____
- Insomnia _____
- Dizziness/loss of balance _____
- Pressure above ears, feeling of head swelling _____
- Sinus problems, tenderness of cheekbones or forehead _____
- Tendency to bruise easily _____
- Eczema, itching eyes _____
- Psoriasis _____
- Chronic hives (urticaria) _____
- Indigestion or heartburn _____
- Sensitivity to milk, wheat, corn or other common foods _____
- Mucus in stools _____
- Rectal itching _____
- Dry mouth or throat _____
- Mouth rashes, including "white" tongue _____
- Bad breath _____
- Foot, hair or body odor not relieved by washing _____
- Nasal congestion or postnasal drip _____
- Nasal itching _____
- Sore throat _____
- Laryngitis, loss of voice _____
- Cough or recurrent bronchitis _____
- Pain or tightness in chest _____
- Wheezing or shortness of breath _____
- Urinary frequency or urgency _____
- Burning on urination _____
- Spots in front of eyes or erratic vision _____
- Burning or tearing eyes _____
- Recurrent infections or fluid in ears _____
- Ear pain or deafness _____

Total Score, Section C _____

Grand Total (Sections A, B and C) _____

30

The Grand Total score will help you and your physician decide if your health problems are yeast-connected. Scores in women will run higher, as seven items in the questionnaire apply exclusively to women, while only two apply exclusively to men.

- Yeast-connected health problems are *almost certainly* present in women with scores of more than 180, and in men with scores of more than 140.
- Yeast-connected health problems are *probably present* in women with scores of more than 120, and in men with scores more than 90.
- Yeast-connected health problems are *possibly present* in women with scores more than 60, and in men with scores of more than 40.
- With scores of less than 60 in women and 40 in men, yeasts are less apt to be the cause of health problems.

Score of 60-99: *yeast a possible cause of health problems.*
Score of 100-139: *yeast a probable cause of health problems.*
Score of 140 or more: *yeast almost certainly a cause of health problems.*

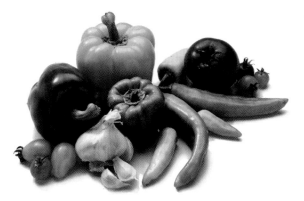

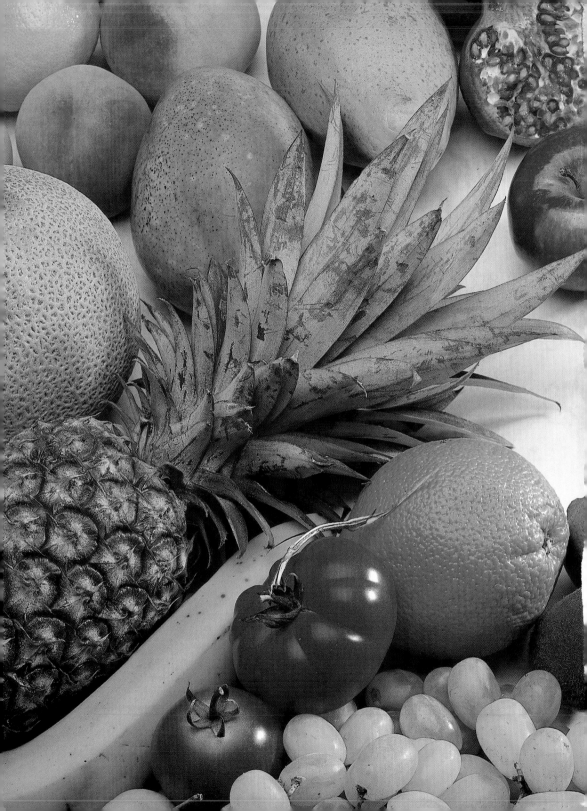

Anti-Candida Recipes

Diet plays a large role in the development of Candida, and will therefore play a large role in recovery.

Papaya and Grapefruit with Kamut®

½ **papaya**

½ **grapefruit**

1 **cup** (150 g) **unsweetened Kamut® flakes**

½ **cup** (125 ml) **freshly squeezed orange juice**

Cut the papaya into ½" (1 cm) cubes (after removing the skin and seeds). Peel and segment the grapefruit. In a large bowl, thoroughly combine the fruit, Kamut® and juice. Serve immediately.

Serves 1

Millet Puffs with Fruit

¼ **cup** (100 g) **fresh strawberries**

¼ **cup** (120 g) **fresh papaya, cut in ½"** (1 cm) **cubes**

½ **banana, sliced**

¼ **cup** (120 g) **fresh grapefruit segments**

½ **cup** (120 g) **millet puffs**

In a bowl, thoroughly combine the fresh fruit and millet puffs.

Serves 1

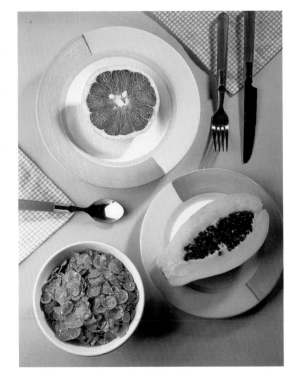

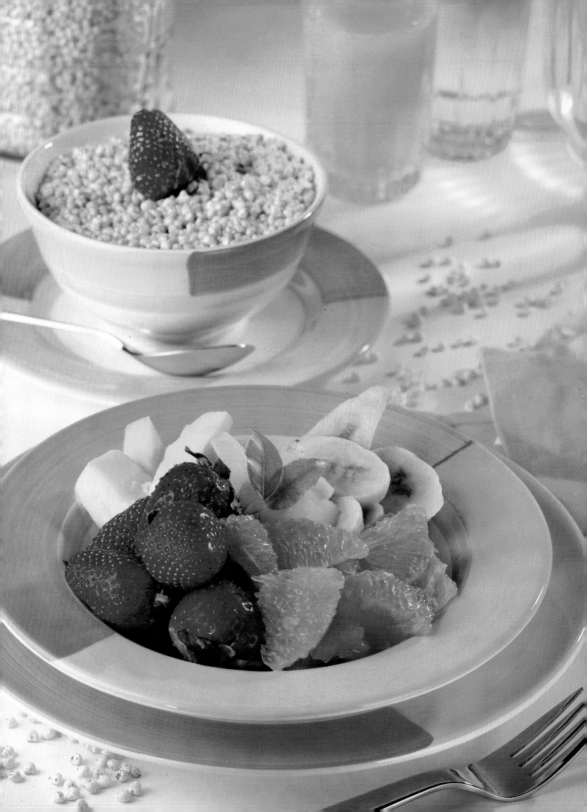

Anti-Candida Salad

2 tbsp apple cider vinegar

I piece whole clove

**I small piece
    cinnamon stick**

**I medium red beet,
    peeled and cut into
    ½" (I cm) chunks**

I bay leaf

½ lemon

**¼ cup (120 g) pumpkin,
    cut into chunks**

**I heart of romaine
    lettuce, leaves separated**

**I medium apple, peeled
    and cut into chunks**

**¼ cup (100 g) toasted
    walnut pieces**

Dressing:

**3 tbsp freshly squeezed
    lemon juice**

**4 tbsp cold-pressed
    flax seed oil**

**I tsp fresh tarragon,
    chopped**

½ tsp honey

**Sea salt or Herbamare
    and freshly ground
    pepper, to taste**

In a large pot, combine 2 quarts (2 l) water, apple cider vinegar, cloves and cinnamon and bring to a boil. Add the beets, cover and simmer for 25 minutes or until tender. Drain and let cool. You can cook the beets a day ahead if you wish.

In a medium pot, combine 1 quart (1 l) water, ½ lemon, and one bay leaf. Bring to a boil. Add the pumpkin and cook for 10 minutes. Remove lemon and bay leaf.

In a large bowl, thoroughly combine beet, pumpkin, lettuce, apple and walnuts.

In a separate bowl, whisk the dressing ingredients together. Pour dressing over the salad and serve immediately.

Serves 2

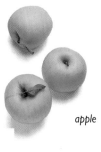

apple

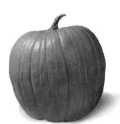

pumpkin

Herbamare is a seasoning made with sea salt and 14 organic herbs. The special steeping process used to make this natural product allows the full herb and vegetable flavor to become concentrated in the salt crystal–preserving essential vitamins and minerals and providing ultimate zest.

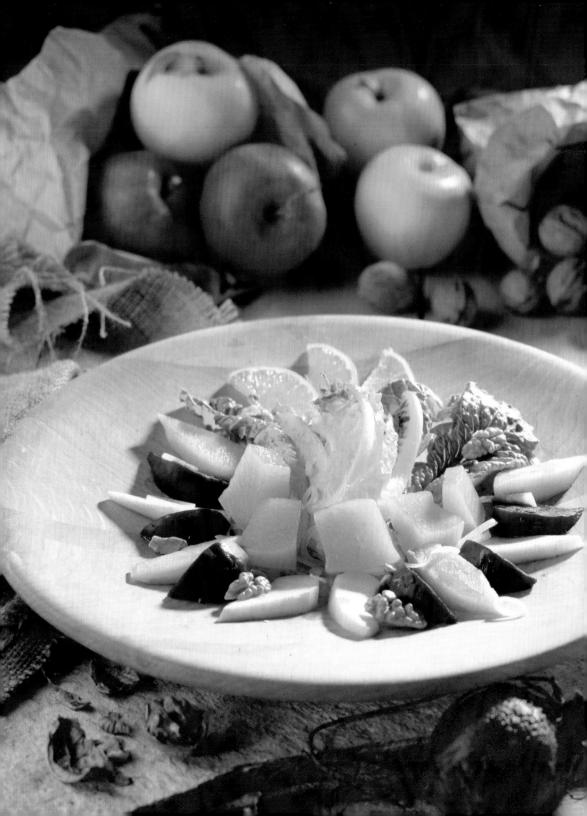

Onion and Tomato Salad

This anti-candida recipe looks great and tastes even better. It makes an impressive salad for guests.

½ cup (200 g) snow peas

1 large beefsteak tomato, sliced

1 medium Bermuda onion, sliced

Dressing:

4 tbsp cold-pressed hazelnut or flax oil

3 tbsp freshly squeezed lemon or lime juice

1 tsp fresh rosemary, chopped

Sea salt and freshly ground pepper, to taste

In a pot, bring 2 quarts (2 l) of water to a boil, add the snow peas and blanch for 2 minutes. Drain and rinse in ice water immediately. In a bowl, whisk oil, lemon juice, rosemary, salt and pepper together. In a separate large bowl, toss the tomato, onion and snow peas with the dressing and serve immediately.

Serves 2

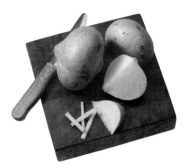

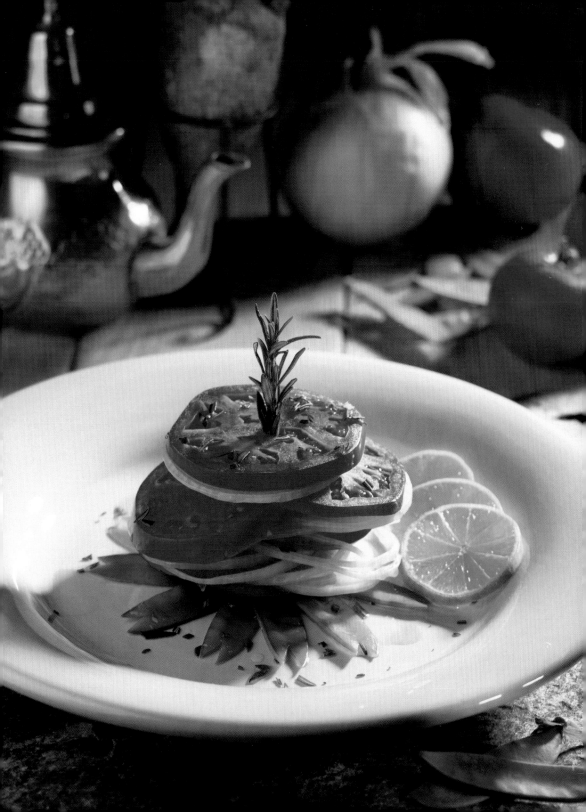

Magnificent Red Beet Soup

This marvellous soup can be served hot or cold.

- **I lb (450 g) red beets, peeled and cut into chunks**
- **I tbsp apple cider vinegar**
- **Pinch ground cloves**
- **½ cinnamon stick**
- **3 tbsp extra-virgin olive oil**
- **I medium shallot, minced**
- **I clove garlic**
- **¼ cup (100 g) celery, diced**
- **¼ cup (100 g) carrot, diced**
- **I tbsp butter**
- **Pinch ground nutmeg**
- **Sea salt and freshly ground pepper, to taste**
- **Whipping cream or kefir for garnish**

In a large pot, combine 2 quarts (2 l) water, vinegar, cloves and cinnamon. Bring to a boil. Add beets, cover and simmer for 45 minutes or until tender. Drain and save the liquid. Remove cinnamon stick.

In a second large pot, heat the oil over medium heat and sauté the shallot, garlic, celery and carrot until translucent. Add the cooked beets, butter, maple syrup, spices and nutmeg. Sauté for 1 to 2 minutes. Add the reserved beet juice, cover and simmer for 5 minutes.

In a blender, mix until very smooth. Serve with a tablespoon of whipping cream or kefir.

Serves 2

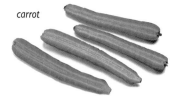

carrot

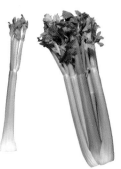

celery

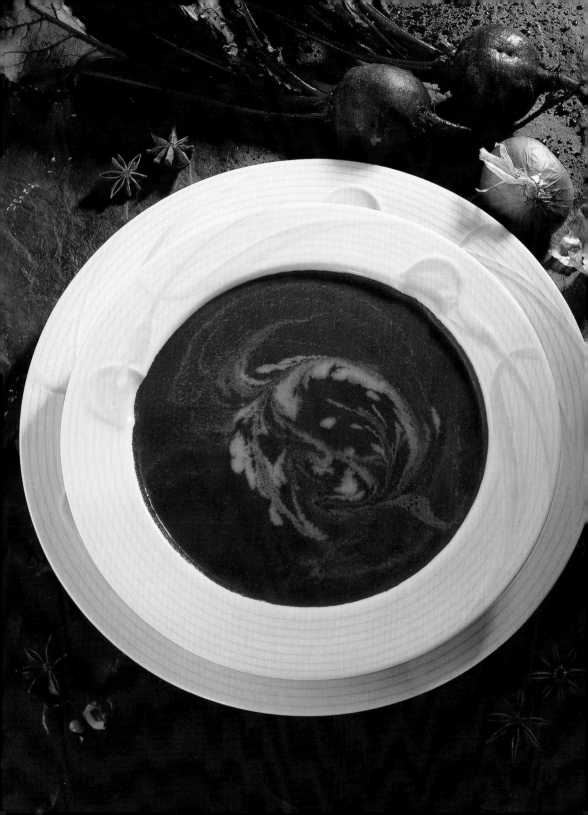

Cucumber-Avocado Soup

Simple, fast and tasty! This is especially wonderful when served cold on a hot summer day.

1 ripe avocado, cut in small chunks

2 cloves garlic, minced

1 shallot, minced

½ English cucumber, grated

1 cup (450 ml) **kefir or goat's milk yogurt**

¼ cup (250 ml) **sparkling water**

1 tbsp lime juice

2 tbsp cold-pressed hazelnut, walnut or flax oil

Fresh herbs of your choice (parsley, dill, tarragon, thyme)

Pinch ground nutmeg

Sea salt and freshly ground pepper, to taste

In a large bowl, thoroughly combine all ingredients, making sure the cucumber is not too watery. Cover and refrigerate at least 1 hour before serving.

Serves 2

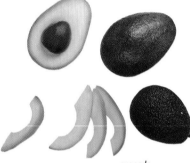

avocado

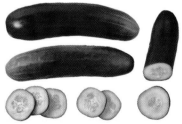

cucumber

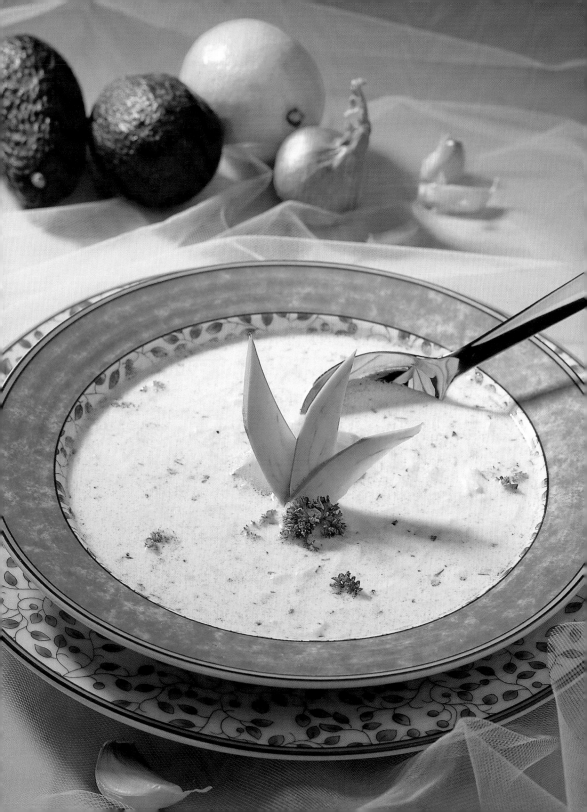

Vegetable Festival

1 cup (150 g) **broccoli florettes**

1 cup (100 g) **Brussels sprouts**

½ lb (225 g) **whole asparagus**

1 large **red bell pepper**

1 large **yellow bell pepper**

½ lb (225 g) **medium eggplant, cut in ¼" slices**

1 small **zucchini, cut in ¼" slices**

1 cup **leeks** (white parts only) **cut lengthwise in half and in 2½" (6 cm) pieces**

¼ cup (100 g) **garlic cloves**

½ cup (125 ml) **extra-virgin olive oil**

Dressing:

2 tbsp **apple cider vinegar or lavender vinegar**

2 tbsp **freshly squeezed lemon juice**

4 tbsp **cold-pressed pumpkin or flax seed oil**

Sea salt and freshly ground pepper, to taste

Fresh herbs for garnish (sage or oregano)

Preheat oven to 375°F (190°C).

In a large pot, bring 2 quarts (2 l) of water to a boil and blanch the broccoli florettes, Brussels sprouts and asparagus for 2 to 3 minutes. Drain the vegetables and immediately rinse with ice water to maintain the rich colors and to keep them crunchy. Set aside.

Wash peppers, cut them in half and remove the seeds. Place the peppers, eggplant, zucchini, leeks and garlic on a cookie sheet and brush both sides of the vegetables with oil. Place in the oven and roast, turning once, until both sides are golden brown (approximately 10 minutes).

Place the peppers in a bowl, cover and set aside. Once cool, carefully peel the skin off the peppers.

In the meantime, whisk all the dressing ingredients together.

Arrange the vegetables on a platter, drizzle dressing over top and serve immediately.

Serves 2

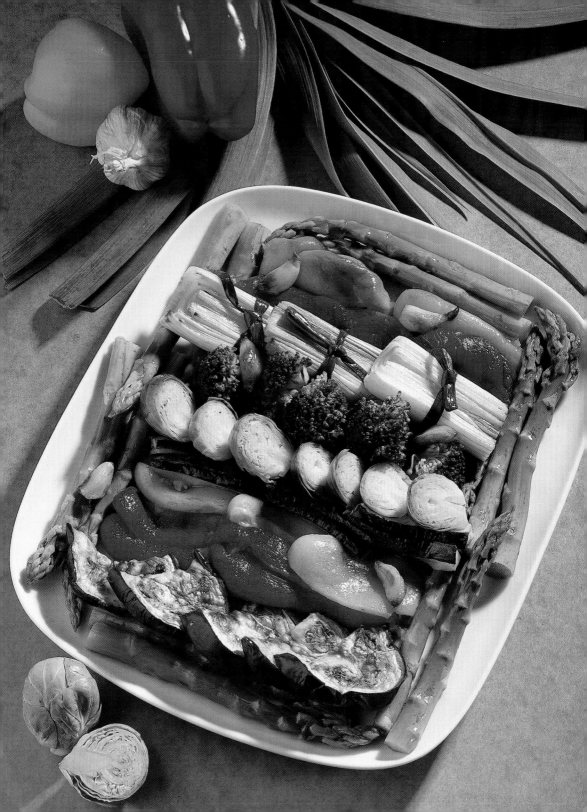

Winter Vegetables with Tofu

Organic vegetables are tasty allies in the fight against candida. This satisfying recipe is a favorite—even with those who are not attempting to control yeast.

- **1 medium kohlrabi**
- **1 medium yam**
- **1 small carrot**
- **1 cup broccoli florettes**
- **2 tbsp coconut butter**
- **½ lb (200 g) firm tofu** (organic, fermented), **cut in 1" (2.5 cm) chunks**
- **1 tbsp garlic, minced**
- **1 tbsp ginger, minced**
- **2 tbsp freshly squeezed lemon juice**
- **1 tbsp butter**
- **1 tsp toasted sesame oil**
- **1 tsp fresh tarragon, chopped**
- **Sea salt and freshly ground pepper, to taste**

Peel and cut the kohlrabi, yam and carrot into 1" (2.5 cm) chunks. Steam the vegetables (a bamboo steamer works well) adding them to the steamer in the following order: kohlrabi first, yam and carrot next, and then broccoli. Steam until tender.

Meanwhile in a large saucepan, heat the coconut butter on medium heat then sauté the tofu until golden. Add garlic and ginger and sauté again. Add lemon juice and butter. Simmer for 1 minute. Stir in sesame oil and tarragon.

Arrange the tofu and vegetables on a platter, pour the sauce over top and serve immediately.

Serves 2

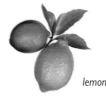

lemon

broccoli

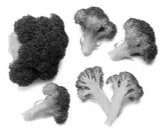

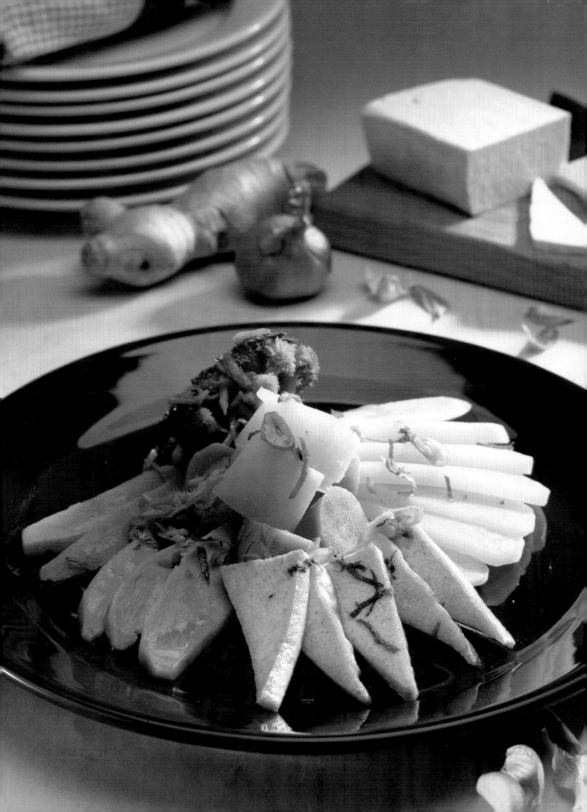

Savoy Cabbage with Baked Potato

2 large Yukon gold
potatoes

Cabbage rolls:

4 large Savoy cabbage
leaves

I cup (150 g) Savoy
cabbage, julienned

2 tbsp extra-virgin
olive oil

3 cloves garlic, minced

I large red bell pepper,
julienned

I large yellow bell pepper,
julienned

½ lb (225 g) asparagus,
julienned

I medium turnip,
julienned

I small white onion,
julienned

4 tbsp butter

½ tbsp freshly squeezed
lemon juice

I tbsp fresh oregano,
chopped

Pinch ground cinnamon

Pinch ground paprika

¼ cup (125 ml) vegetable stock

Sea salt and freshly ground pepper
(preferably lemon pepper), to taste

Preheat oven to 375°F (190°C).

To prepare the baked potatoes, carefully wash and dry them and brush with oil. Wrap each in foil and bake for 45 minutes or until soft. Remove and set aside. Set aside 2 tablespoon of your butter to put on potatoes when serving. Reduce the oven temperature to 275°F (135°C).

While your potato is baking, prepare the cabbage rolls. Bring 2 quarts (2 l) of water, with ½ tablespoon of salt, to a boil and blanch the cabbage leaves for 3 minutes. Drain and cool in ice water then cut out the middle part of the stem, leaving the leaves whole.

In a large saucepan, heat the oil on medium heat and sauté the remaining vegetables for 5 to 6 minutes. Add butter, lemon juice, oregano, spices, and cook until tender. Season with salt and pepper.

To assemble, divide the vegetables (approximately 2 to 3 tablespoons per leaf) and place each portion onto a cabbage leaf. Tightly roll the leaves, tucking in the ends as you roll. Place in the oven for 10 minutes. Serve with the baked potatoes.

Serves 2

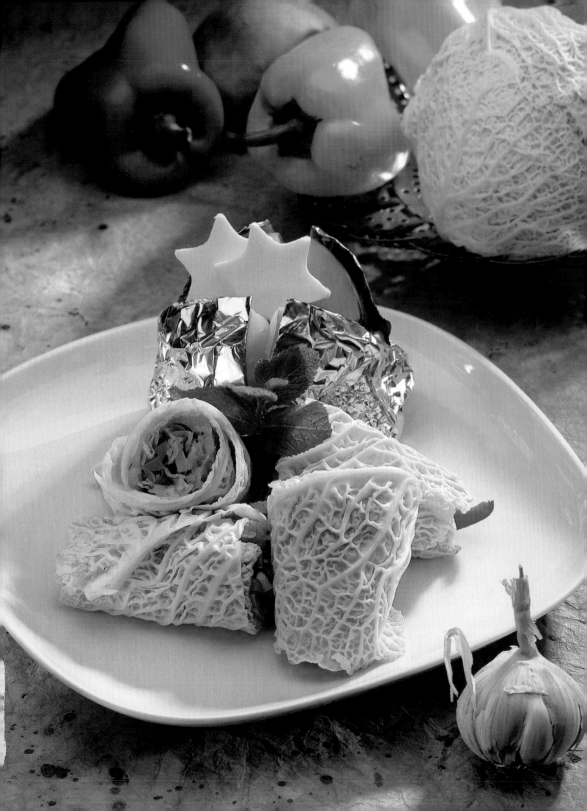

Baked Seasonal Vegetables

This tower of nutrition is a fun way to regain health and vigor.

½ lb asparagus, cut in 2"
(5 cm) **pieces**

I **large zucchini, cut in** ¼"
(5 mm) **slices**

I **large eggplant, cut in** ½"
(5 mm) **slices**

I **large red bell pepper,
cut in half**

I **large yellow bell pepper,
cut in half**

I **large red onion, sliced**

I **large beefsteak tomato,
cut in half**

I **2"-piece leek, cut in half**

4 tbsp extra-virgin
olive oil

Sea salt and freshly
ground pepper, to taste

Dressing:

I tbsp freshly squeezed
lemon juice

I tsp fresh thyme,
chopped

I tbsp cold-pressed
flax seed oil

Sea salt and Herbamare,
to taste

Preheat oven to 375°F (190°C).

In a large pot, bring 2 quarts (2 l) of water, with 1 tablespoon of salt, to a boil and blanch the asparagus for 3 to 4 minutes or until tender. Drain, cool with ice water and set aside.

Brush remaining vegetables with olive oil, season with salt and pepper, and place on a cookie sheet. Place in the oven and bake, turning once, until both sides are golden brown (approximately 10 minutes).

Meanwhile, whisk all dressing ingredients together in a bowl.

Place the baked vegetables in the center of each plate and arrange the asparagus around them. Drizzle the dressing over top and serve immediately.

Serves 2

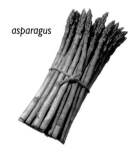

asparagus

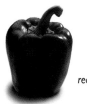

red pepper

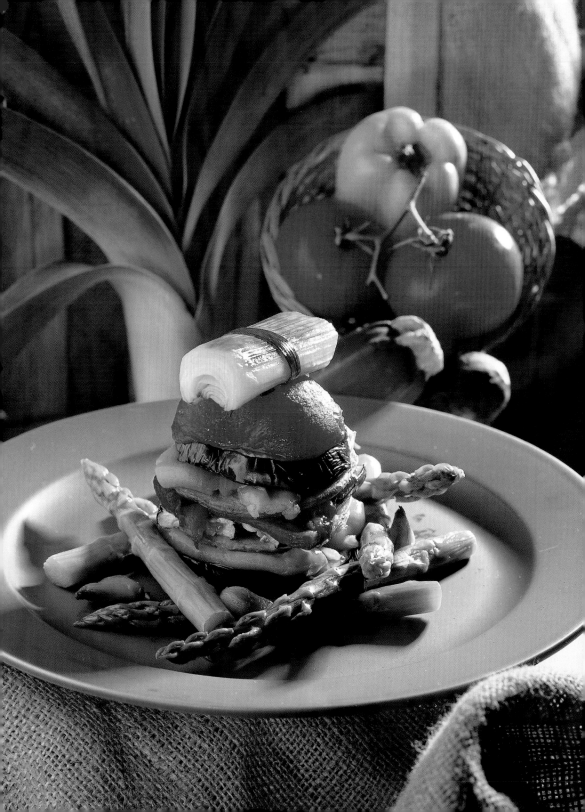

Avocado Salad

The avocado is an amazing food—high in protein, vitamins and minerals. This salad is so satisfying, you may call it dinner.

1 large avocado

8 asparagus tips

1 ripe tomato, sliced

Sea salt and freshly ground pepper, to taste

Avocado-Mayonnaise Dressing:

2 large egg yolks

2 tbsp white wine or apple cider vinegar

1 tsp Dijon mustard

1 tbsp lemon or lime juice

1 to 2 drops Worcestershire sauce

1 to 2 drops Tabasco sauce

1½ cup (375 ml) pure olive or flax oil

Sea salt and Herbamare, to taste

½ ripe avocado, puréed

To prepare the dressing, beat together the egg yolks, vinegar and mustard in a large bowl until light-colored and smooth. Add the lemon juice, Worcestershire and Tabasco and beat again.

While beating, add half the oil, a few drops at a time. As the mixture starts to thicken, slowly add the rest of the oil. Continue beating until the mayonnaise becomes thick. Purée the avocado and add it to the mayonnaise. Season with salt and pepper. Set aside.

To prepare the vegetables, bring 2 quarts (2 l) of water with 1 tablespoon of salt to a boil in a large pot. Blanch the asparagus for 3 to 4 minutes or until tender. Drain, cool with ice water and set aside.

Cut the avocado into thin slices.

Using a squeeze bottle, squeeze the avocado-mayonnaise into a checker board pattern onto plates. Arrange the avocado on top in a fan shape and garnish with the tomato and asparagus. Season with salt and freshly ground pepper and serve immediately.

Serves 2

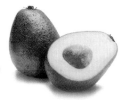

avocado

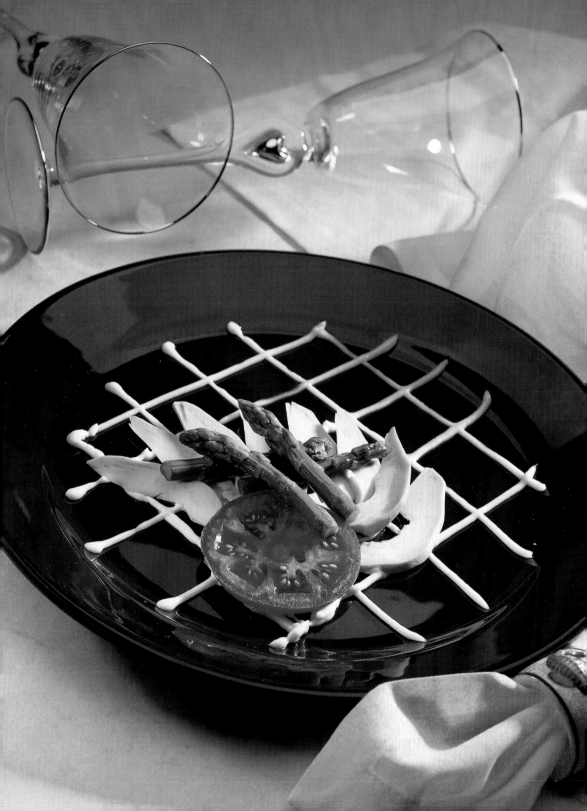

Colorful Kohlrabi and Beet Soup

This exquisite looking soup calls for a special evening of yeast fighting.

4 (1lb or 450 g) medium red beets, cooked

1 tbsp apple cider vinegar

Pinch ground cloves

1 cinnamon stick

1 lb (450 g) kohlrabi, cooked

2 tbsp extra-virgin olive oil

2 medium shallots, minced

2 cloves garlic, minced

1½ cups (375 ml) vegetable stock

1 cup (250 ml) cream

Herbamare, to taste

1 tbsp cold-pressed flax seed oil, for garnish

In a large pot, combine 2 quarts (2 l) water, vinegar, cloves and ½ stick of cinnamon. Bring to a boil. Add the beets, cover and simmer for 45 minutes or until tender. Drain and set aside.

In a medium pot, combine 1 quart (1 l) of water, 1 bay leaf, ½ stick of cinnamon and one teaspoon of salt. Bring to boil and add kohlrabi. Cook for 15 minutes or until tender.

In a pot, heat 1 tablespoon of oil over medium heat and sauté half the shallots and half the garlic until golden brown. Add the red beet, half the vegetable stock, and half the cream. Cover and simmer until the liquid is reduced by half.

In a separate pot repeat the above paragraph with the cooked kohlrabi.

Blend the soups in a blender (separately) until they become the same consistency. Season the soups with salt and pepper.

Pour both soups at the same time into soup bowls. Because of their similar consistencies, each soup will stay separate. Drizzle flax seed oil over top and serve immediately.

Serves 2

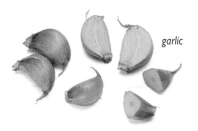

garlic

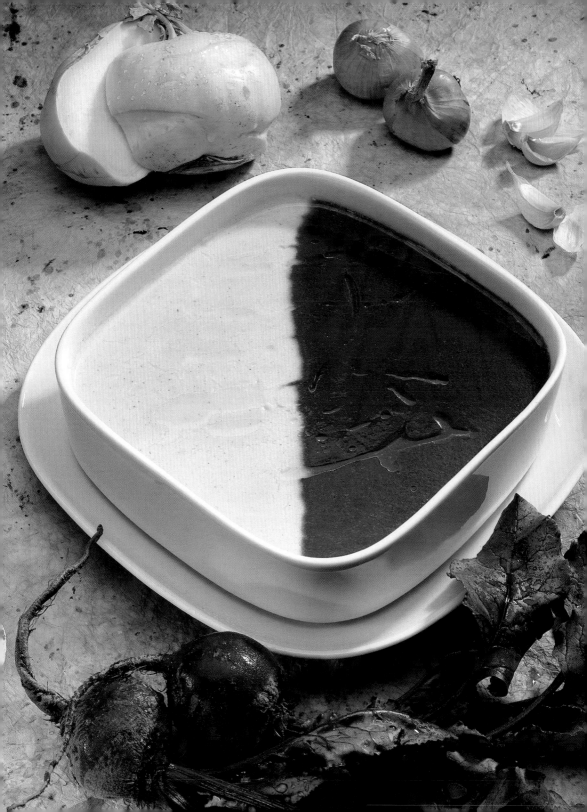

Potato Soup

This satisfying and tasty soup is "comfort food" at its best.

1 lb russet potatoes, peeled

2 tbsp extra-virgin olive oil

1 small white onion, diced

4 cloves garlic, minced

2 cups (450 ml) **vegetable stock**

2 bay leaves

¼ cup (60 ml) **cream**

Pinch nutmeg

Herbamare, to taste

Fresh parsley, for garnish

In a pot, boil the potatoes in 1½ quarts (1½ l) water, with 1 teaspoon of salt, until done. Drain carefully, reserving the liquid, and set aside.

Meanwhile, in another pot, heat the oil over medium heat and sauté the onion and garlic until translucent. Add vegetable stock, bay leaves, cream, nutmeg, salt and pepper. Cover and bring to a boil then cook for 4 to 5 minutes more. Slowly add cooked potatoes one after the other to control consistency (should be creamy) and cook 5 to 7 minutes more.

Remove the bay leaves then blend with a hand mixer. If the consistency is too thick (it should be like honey) add a little bit of the reserved potato water and blend again. Garnish with parsley and serve immediately.

Serves 2

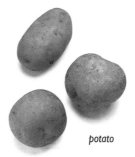

potato

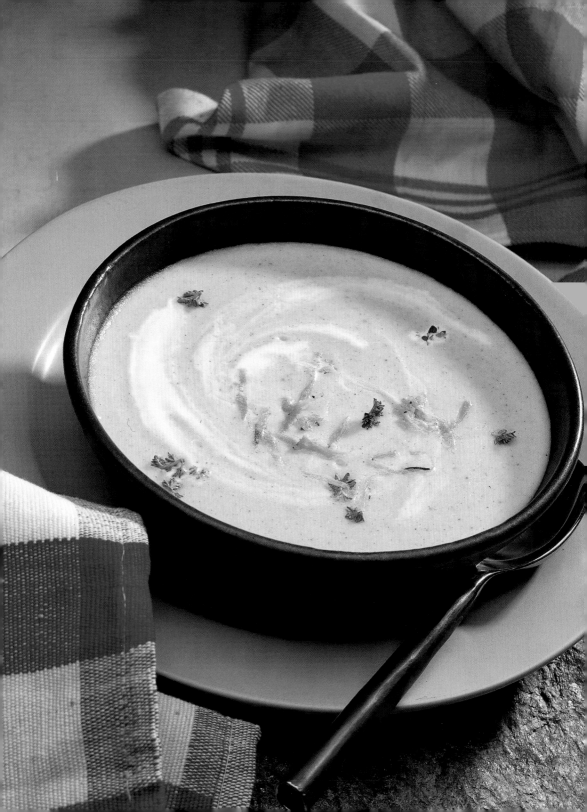

Tomato-Tofu Tower

Who said yeast busting had to be dull? This exciting dish is impressive to both the eyes and taste buds.

½ lb (250 g) **firm tofu** (organic, fermented), **cut into** ¼" (5 mm) **slices**

I large **beefsteak tomato,** **cut into** ¼" (5 mm) **slices**

I lb (450 g) **asparagus,** **cut in** 3" (7.5 cm) **pieces**

Marinade:

I tbsp **toasted sesame oil**

I tbsp **freshly squeezed lemon juice**

I tbsp **rice wine**

I tbsp **sweet cherry balsamic vinegar**

2 tbsp **cold-pressed pumpkin seed oil**

2 cloves **garlic, minced**

I small **shallot, minced**

I tbsp **chopped fresh cilantro**

Zest of one lemon

Herbamare, to taste

In a bowl, whisk together all the marinade ingredients until the mixture emulsifies. Pour the mixture over the tofu, cover and refrigerate overnight.

To prepare the tomato-tofu towers, stack the tomato and marinated tofu in alternating layers. Reserve the marinade. Tie the asparagus around the towers with a straw string. Place in a steamer (a bamboo steamer works well) and steam for 7 to 10 minutes at medium heat.

Carefully remove the towers and place them onto plates. Pour the remaining marinade over top and serve immediately.

Serves 2

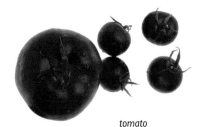

tomato

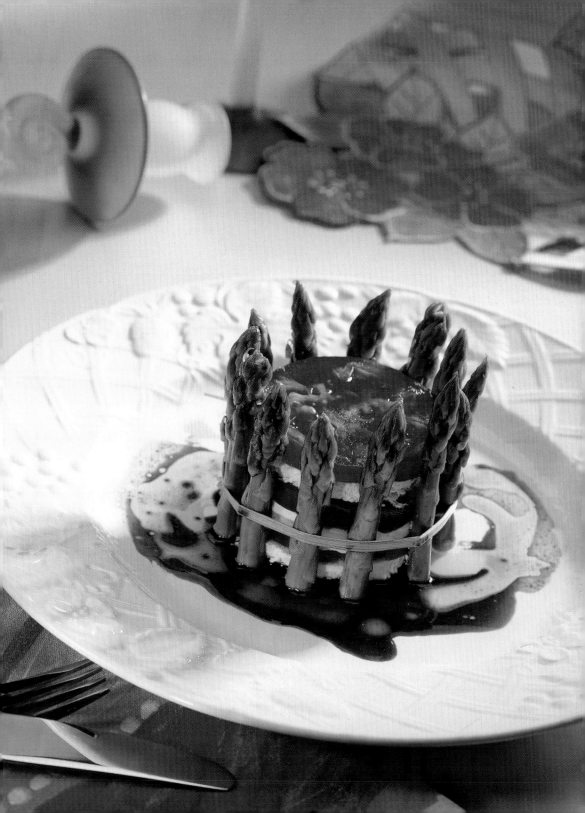

Quinoa-Vegetable Patties

I cup (180 g) **quinoa**

I cup (150 g) **carrots, finely grated**

I medium **onion, diced**

½ tsp **Herbamare**

I tbsp **Braggs all-purpose seasoning**

I tbsp **tomato paste**

I free-range **egg**

½ cup (100 g) **bread crumbs**

½ cup (100 g) **sunflower seeds, finely chopped**

½ cup (100 g) **walnuts, shelled and coarsely chopped**

½ tsp **fresh thyme, chopped**

½ tsp **ground coriander**

Pinch **ground cumin**

I tsp **ginger, minced**

⅓ cup (85 ml) **coconut oil**

I tsp **garlic, minced**

½ cup (120 g) **zucchini, grated**

½ cup (120 g) **pumpkin** (or spaghetti squash), **grated**

I tbsp **fresh cilantro, chopped**

Sea salt and Herbamare, to taste

In a pot, cook the quinoa in 1 quart (1 l) of salted water for 15 minutes. Set aside to cool.

Meanwhile, in a large bowl, combine the carrots, half the onion, Herbamare, Braggs seasoning, tomato paste, egg, bread crumbs, walnuts and sunflower seeds. Add the thyme, coriander and cumin and mix thoroughly. Add cooked quinoa.

In a pan, heat 1 tablespoon of coconut oil at medium heat and sauté the ginger, garlic, remaining onion, zucchini and pumpkin until translucent. Add cilantro, salt and pepper and mix thoroughly. To make a patty, take 1 handful of the mixture and shape it into a ball. With the thumb make a hole in the center and place 1 tablespoon of the vegetable mixture into the hole.

Roll the dough carefully until the vegetable doesn't show anymore, then flatten into a patty.

Heat the remaining coconut oil and sauté the patties for 4 to 5 minutes on each side. Serve with a fresh salad of your choice.

Serves 2

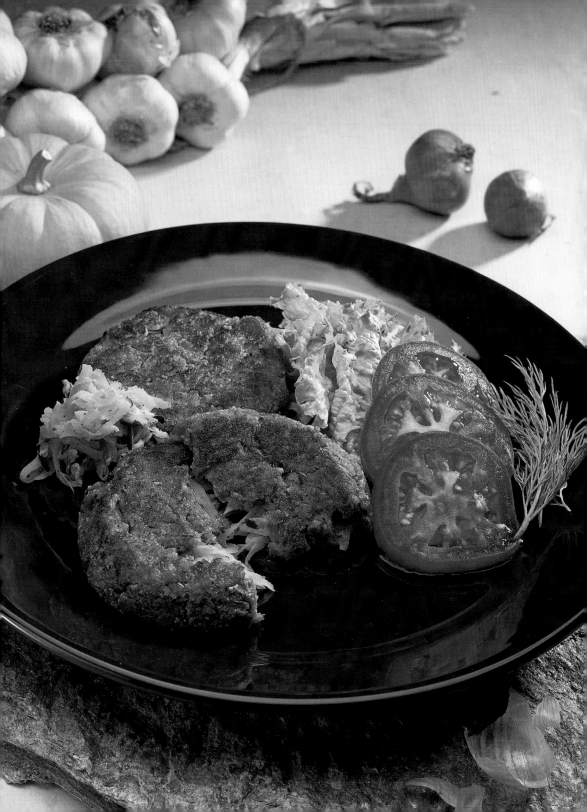

Vegetable Medley with Poached Egg

2 tbsp apple cider vinegar

½ tbsp sea salt

2 bay leaves

1 tsp coriander seeds

2 whole cloves

1 fennel bulb, sliced

4 baby carrots, sliced

1 red bell pepper,
   quartered

1 yellow bell pepper,
   quartered

3 tbsp extra-virgin
   olive oil

1 tbsp butter

1 small white onion,
   julienned

1 clove garlic, minced

1½ cups (300 g) endive

1 large egg, poached

Dressing:

2 tbsp extra-virgin olive oil

2 tbsp cold-pressed
   flax seed oil

1 tsp freshly squeezed
   lemon juice

1 tbsp fresh parsley, chopped

1 dash Maggi or Bragg's aminos

1 dash Herbamare, to taste

In a large pot, combine 1 quart (1 l) of water, apple cider vinegar and salt. Bring to a boil. Add bay leaves, coriander and cloves. Blanch the fennel, carrots and peppers for 4 to 5 minutes. Drain, rinse with ice water and set aside.

Meanwhile, whisk all dressing ingredients together in a bowl.

In a pan, heat the olive oil and butter over medium heat and sauté the onion and garlic for 4 to 5 minutes or until translucent. Add the endive and sauté lightly for 30 seconds.

Arrange the endive, fennel, carrots and peppers on a plate. Drizzle the dressing over top and serve with a poached egg.

Serves 1

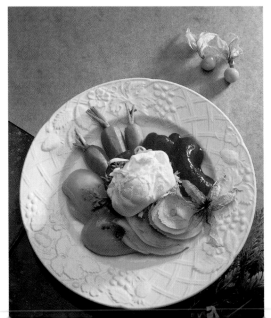

references

Bennett, J. E. "Searching for the yeast connection."
New England Journal of Medicine.
Vol. 323 (1990): 176-67.

Haas, E. M. Staying Healthy with Nutrition.
Berkeley: Celestial Arts, 1992.

Zwerling, M. H., K. N. Owens, and N. H. Ruth. 1984.
"Think yeast: The expanding spectrum of
candidiasis." South Carolina Med. Assoc.
Vol. 80 (1984): 454-456.

Skolnick, A. "Even air in the home is not
entirely free of potential pollutants: Medical news and
perspectives." JAMA. Vol. 262 (1989): 3102-3103,
3107.

sources

for Herbamare:
Bioforce
4001 Cote Verty
Saint Laurent H4R 1R5
Tel: (514) 335-9393
Fax: (514) 335-9639

Rapunzel Pure Organics
2424 State Route
203 Valatia 12184 USA
Tel: 1-800-207-2814
Tel: (518) 392-8620
Fax: (518) 392-8630
email: mkg@rapunzel.com

for Yeast Buster kit:
Innovite
97 Saramia Crescent
Concord, ON L4K 4P7
Tel: (905) 761-5121
Fax: (905) 761-1453

for natural oils:
Flora
7400 Fraser Park Drive
Burnaby, BC V5J 5B9
(604) 436-6000
1-800-663-0617 (Western Canada)
1-800-387-7541 (Eastern Canada)

Flora Inc.
P.O. Box 73
Lynden, WA
98264
(360) 354-2110

First published in 2000 by
alive books
7436 Fraser Park Drive
Burnaby BC V5J 5B9
(604) 435-1919
1-800–661–0303

© 2000 by **alive books**

Artwork:
  Terence Yeung
  Raymond Cheung
  Liza Novecoski
  Paul Chau
Food Styling/Recipe Development:
  Fred Edrissi
Photographs:
  Edmond Fong (recipe photos)
  Siegfried Gursche
Photo Editing:
  Sabine Edrissi-Bredenbrock
Editing:
  Sandra Tonn
  Marian MacLean

Canadian Cataloguing in
Publication Data

Crook, William G.
  Nature's Own Candida Cure

(**alive** natural health guides, 8
ISSN 1490-6503)
ISBN 1-55312-002-7
Second printing, 2000

Printed in Canada

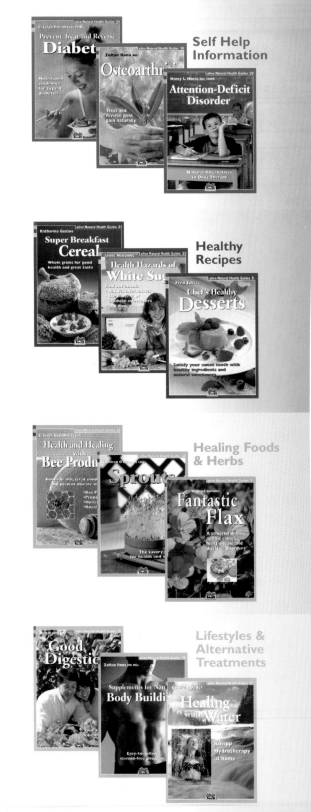